Bodyweight Training For Beginners:

Bodyweight Training Guide

By

Charles Maldonado

Table of Contents

Introduction 5

Chapter 1. What are Bodyweight Exercises? 7

Chapter 2. Benefits of Bodyweight Exercises 8

Chapter 3. Types of Bodyweight Exercises 13

    Common Core Bodyweight Exercises 13

    Common Lower Body Bodyweight Exercises 18

    Common Upper Bodyweight Exercises 22

Chapter 4. A Basic Bodyweight Training Plan for Beginners 24

Thank You Page 30

Bodyweight Training For Beginners: Bodyweight Training Guide

By Charles Maldonado

© Copyright 2014 Charles Maldonado

Reproduction or translation of any part of this work beyond that permitted by section 107 or 108 of the 1976 United States Copyright Act without permission of the copyright owner is unlawful. Requests for permission or further information should be addressed to the author.

This publication is designed to provide accurate and authoritative information in regard to the subject matter covered. This work is sold with the understanding that the publisher is not engaged in rendering legal, accounting, or other professional services. If legal advice or other expert assistance is required, the services of a competent professional person should be sought.

First Published, 2014

Printed in the United States of America

Introduction

For many people who want to look younger, have more energy, and have the possibility of living longer and healthier, engaging in a regular exercise program provides unequalled benefits that can be both seen and felt. Whether you are a man or woman, anyone can reap the healthy benefits that exercise provides. Regular exercise helps control weight and can help you fight conditions such as heart disease and bad cholesterol. Regular exercise also helps you improve your mood and provides you with sustainable energy that can help you power through your day.

While exercise itself can be a fun and enjoyable activity, many beginners are hesitant to start an exercise program or may lack the motivation in finding a program that will work best for their needs. Gym memberships can be costly and they may feel lost in the crowd amidst the rows of workout machines and countless people. While there are many fitness and exercise programs that are available for purchase on DVD, these can also be costly and involve extra equipment that needs to be bought. For beginners who are looking to start reaping the excellent benefits of exercise and are able to do it in the comfort of their home for little to no money, a bodyweight exercise program is the perfect solution.

Chapter 1. What are Bodyweight Exercises?

Bodyweight exercises are the most common and basic exercises that people can do in order to build strength and stamina. With bodyweight exercises, men and women are using the weight of their own bodies and don't need to use machines or equipment. Because the apparatus in your body, bodyweight exercises are the ultimate in convenience and portability and you can perform these types of exercises in your home, hotel room and even your office. When done correctly and with variety, basic movements such as push-ups, chin-ups, and sit-ups can provide men and women with an efficient workout that can be done anytime and anywhere.

Chapter 2. Benefits of Bodyweight Exercises

For many of those who are starting their journey on the road to fitness, they may find it hard to believe that it is possible to sculpt a lean and toned body without the use of free weights and other workout machines. A main reason why many beginners may be hesitant in starting a workout program or may abandon a program after a short period of time is the fact they feel exercise is like rocket science and need to follow a complex set of exercises. Bodyweight exercises are an excellent choice for beginners to build the strength they desire while building muscle and improving their cardiovascular health. The following are some benefits of bodyweight exercises that may them great for beginners, as well as all exercise enthusiasts:

Bodyweight Exercises are Efficient

Because there is no equipment that needs to be used, bodyweight exercises are extremely efficient and people can quickly move from one exercise to another after a short rest period. Additionally, because of these quick transitions and shorter rest periods, people can raise their heart rate and burn calories faster.

You Get Two Main Benefits for the Price of One

The two main goals of any exercise program is to build strength and increase cardiovascular fitness. Bodyweight exercises are able to provide both benefits in a workout program that can benefit anybody, even if time is short. For example, exercisers can perform a series of push-ups then in the next exercise perform a set of jumping jacks then follow it with a set of walking lunges. With the great variety of exercises that are possible with bodyweight training, people can easily mix and match their exercises and workout.

Bodyweight Exercises are Easy to Modify

No matter what the age or fitness level, bodyweight exercises can be modified to fit anyone. For example, beginners can start off with exercises with low repetitions and can increase those repetitions as they begin to build strength. People can also vary the difficulty of their workouts by performing exercises at a slower pace, and by perform exercises with perfect technique, both men and women are able to change up their intensity and see measurable results.

Body Flexibility

Bodyweight exercises offer men and women a full range of motion that free weights or other machines can't offer. With full of range of motion, joints can move more freely which can lead to improve overall movement and posture. Additionally, exercise which are able to provide full range of motion can reduce workout-related injuries.

No Time? No Sweat!

A common reason (or excuse) that many people use in not utilizing and exercises program is they don't have time. Bodyweight exercises can be performed anywhere and anytime. Additionally, performing these exercises without machines or other equipment can be a great form of stress release that can be done at home, office, hotel room or anywhere else there is space.

Cost

Exercise can have the potential to be an expensive endeavor. Gym memberships and personal trainers can significantly strain household and personal budgets. Bodyweight exercises have become more popular among people of all fitness levels because of their simplicity and there is no need for equipment.

Safety

Arguably, the most common reason why men and women abandon exercise programs is due to injury. While the common saying that *no pain no gain* may hold true in the world of fitness, the aches and pains associated with exercise can turn many people away. Bodyweight exercises are relatively safe for men and women of all fitness levels and experience. In fact, the basic movements of bodyweight exercises can not only prevent injury, but can also be used to rehabilitate any injury.

Bodyweight Exercises are Fun

There are people who feel that exercising indoors can be boring. The beauty of bodyweight exercises is they can be done indoors, outdoors and with a group of friends. While exercising, people can throw in exercises that may seem a bit silly and will help keep the program lighthearted and fun.

Variety

Doing endless repetitions of curls, deadlifts and squats can be monotonous and dull. With bodyweight exercises, there are countless variations to spice up workouts and provide new challenges that can be exciting. With the variety of exercises, bodyweight training can also help break through any plateaus and will help men and women progress.

Bodyweight Exercises Provide Results

Bodyweight exercises are comprised of what are called compound movements, which means that the exercises involve the movement of numerous joints and muscles. Simple exercises such as push-ups and chin-ups are some of the most effective exercises people can do to increase strength.

Chapter 3. Types of Bodyweight Exercises

Bodyweight exercises can be separated according to the body parts and muscle group these exercises target. While these exercises do target specific areas of the body, they can be modified and combined with other exercises for a full-body muscle and cardiovascular workout. These exercises can be made easy for the beginner or more challenging for those who have advanced levels of fitness. With the wide variety of bodyweight exercises, there are limitless combinations of workouts that men and women can employ in their daily routines. The following are some of the many examples of bodyweight exercises people can engage in and enjoy.

Common Core Bodyweight Exercises

Your core is a complex series of muscles that are incorporated in almost every body movement. When men and women work their core, they are working the muscle in the pelvis, abdominal and back. With a strong core it will improve balance and coordination, improve flexibility, will help people breathe better and will help improve overall strength.

1. Planks-this exercise is also called the *hover* and is similar to a push-up in regards to its look. To execute the plank, a person will place their forearms on the ground and place their toes on the floor. The torso must be straight and rigid and the body should form a straight line all the way from the head to the toes with no bending. While the head is relaxing and looking towards the ground, the position is held as long as the proper form is being kept. Planks can be modified by lifting a leg in the air or using an exercise ball in order to increase difficulty and to work different muscle groups.

2. Side Planks—side planks begin with lying on your side and positioning the elbow just under the shoulder. An individual would then left themselves off the floor using their elbow, being sure that both their body remains rigid and stiff. In general, people will hold that rigid position up to a count of ten then may switch sides. As with the regular plank, the side plank can be modified for intensity by lifting the top leg as high as possible. People who perform side planks can opt to use their hand instead of their elbow to prop them up.

3. Push-ups—push-ups are the most basic of exercises, but it quite possibly the best all-around exercise movement for both men and women. When done correctly, push-ups not only effectively work the core, but also the upper body parts such as triceps, shoulders, and the chest. Additionally, properly done push-ups are excellent leg workouts. For the basic push-up, it starts with getting on the floor and positioning the hands slightly wider than the shoulders.

The next step is to raise the toes to keep balanced and must remember to keep their body in a straight line. On the downward motion of the push-up, the abs and core muscles must be tightened by pulling the belly button towards the spine. As they bend people need to remember to inhale when lowering themselves to the ground and exhale when they return to starting position.

To ensure proper technique, the elbows must be at a 90 degree angle when people are at their lowest point in the push-up. As with other bodyweight exercises, people can add element to the push-up to increase strength and intensity. For example, people can do pushups with a table, chair or up against a wall. Additionally, people can use a medicine ball, workout ball or even dumbbells to add more intensity.

4. V-Sits—the V-Sit is an effective core exercise as it works both the inner and outer oblique muscles as well as engages the hip flexors. To perform this exercise, people need to start in a seated position and lift their legs to a 45 degree angle while contracting their core muscles. As the legs are raised, the arms must be placed straight forward and, if possible, be extended towards the shins. While the position is held, good posture must be maintained for proper form. When going back to normal seated position, people should try and hold the position just before the legs and hands make contact with the floor.

5. Back Bends—this exercise is excellent for the gluteus muscles. To start the exercise, people lie flat on their back with hands to the sides, their knees bent and their feet placed flat on the floor or mat. The hips raise to create a straight line from the knees up to the shoulders, keeping in mind to keep the feet under the knees and to tighten both the abdominal and gluteus muscles. For beginners, they should try to hold this

position for 20 seconds. If they are unable to, they should hold the position as long as possible while keeping perfect form. As strength increases, the position can be held for longer periods.

6. Bridge (Single Leg)—the exercise is a variation of the back bend exercise. With the single-leg bridge, people perform the bank bend exercise and will slowly raise a leg as far and high as possible. It is important that the pelvis remains both raised and is level. This exercise can be performed at 20 to 30 seconds per repetition.

7. Crunches—this exercise is similar to a sit-up with the exception of its range of motion. To perform a crunch, a person will lie on their back with their knees bent and their feet planted on the floor. The hands are placed behind the head and they will slowly peel their head and shoulders from the floor. Once the upper part of the back is off the ground, they will slowly work their way back down to the original laying position. Again, as with other bodyweight exercises that target the core, people must engage their core muscles through contracting and pushing to the spine.

Common Lower Body Bodyweight Exercises

1. Wall Sits—in order to perform a wall sit, a person starts by leaning against a wall and will slowly lower themselves until their thighs reach parallel to the ground. In order for this exercise to fully work, a person's knees must be directly above their ankles and the back must be kept straight. If possible, this seated position should be held for one minute. To add difficulty people can hold the seated position for longer periods or can add some bicep curls with dumbbells or household items.

2. Air Squats—stand with feet shoulder-width apart with arms relaxed at the sides of the body and toes pointed outward at a slight angle. While engaging those important core muscles, pull back the shoulders and bend at the knees. As those motions are being performed both the butt and hips are pushed forward. It is important to keep the weight on the heels and try to get the thighs parallel to the ground if possible. With additional strength, people can try to lower their butt to where it sits behind their calves.

3. Lunges—lunges are another basic bodyweight exercise that are excellent in building strength in the leg muscles. People start with their hands placed on their hips and their feet placed shoulder-width apart. With one leg placed forward, people slowly lower themselves until the forward knee is either close to touching the ground or placed at a 90 degree angle. People then return to the starting position, switch legs then repeat the motion.

For variations, people can perform *jump lunges*, where people perform a regular lunge then jump explosively in the air as they switch legs. People can also perform *walking lunges* where they start in normal lunge position with their knees touching or almost making contact with floor. People then alternate legs and bring their alternate leg forward in a walking motion without pause.

4. Single Leg Deadlifts—this exercise starts with a person in a standing position with their feet placed together. The right leg starts to lift slowly and the arms and torso lower. It is important to keep the left leg slightly bent and, if possible, keep the arms close to the floor. To complete the exercise, slowly raise up

back into standing position. This exercise can be scaled to fit beginners with assistance from a chair or bench, and if they aren't available people they can try to lower themselves to the ground as low as possible without discomfort or pain. With increased strength, people can try to lower themselves as close to the ground as possible.

5. Calf Raises—from the standing position, rise up to the front and balls of the toes, while trying to keep the knees straight and the heels off of the floor. While in that apex position, hold as long as possible and slowly return to normal position. To increase range of motion, engage other muscle groups and to add difficulty, using an inclined surface such as steps is beneficial. Additionally, the use of lighter dumbbells or other household items can help increase strength.

6. Quadruped Leg Lifts—with this leg lift variation, people start resting on their hands and knees. While in this position, it is important to keep the back as flat as possible and to engage the core muscles. When ready, raise the left leg (or right leg) straight back until it is at hip level and is parallel to the ground. While balancing, raise the toe of the opposite foot towards the sky

while tightening the abdominal muscles, back and gluteus muscles.

Common Upper Bodyweight Exercises

1. Superman Pose—while lying flat on the stomach, both the arms and legs will be extended. Raise both arms and legs off the ground at the same time. While performing this upper bodyweight exercise it is important to keep the torso still.

2. Reverse Flyes—for this exercise, men and women can use dumbbells, bottles of water or other household items that are small and have some weight. To start the exercise, people will stand up straight and place one foot slightly in front of the other. While the abdominal muscles are engaged and with the palms facing forward, people will bend slightly forward at the waist and extend their arms out to the side while squeezing the shoulder blades.

3. Triceps Dip—using a chair or bench, people will be seating on the ground facing front with their knees slightly bent. They will then grab the edge of the chair or bench and straighten their arms. The arms should be bent at a 90 degree angle while going upward, then straightened on the downward motion. Once strength has been built, men and women can increase the

intensity of this exercise by reach out one arm while lifting the opposite leg.

4. Inchworm—for people performing this exercise, they need to stand as tall as possible and reach towards the floor with their fingertips. Keeping the legs as straight as possible without locking, they can slowly lower the torso and walk their hands forward as they do so. Once people achieve a push-up like position, they can take small steps until their feet and hands meet.

5. Arm Circles—for this exercise people need to extend their arms out from their bodies and perpendicular to their torso. Once this position is achieved people start making small circles, first in a clockwise fashion then counterclockwise. The circles should be about a foot in circumference if able and the rotations should last for at least 20 seconds before rotating.

6. Boxer—this exercise starts with the knees bent and feet placed hip-width apart. People will then keep their elbows tucked in and extend one arm forward in a punching motion. Once the arm comes back into the tucked position the same motion can be done with the other arm.

Chapter 4. A Basic Bodyweight Training Plan for Beginners

For beginners who are starting on the road to fitness and overall wellness, one of the great benefits of engaging in bodyweight training is that you can start as simple and basic as you want. You can do these exercises in the privacy of your own home and can start with just a few basic exercises. As you gain strength and stamina, you can incorporate more exercises in your regimen. Additionally, more moves and variations can be incorporated into basic bodyweight exercises to increase break out of the ruts you may encounter. Additionally, the addition of different variations of exercises will increase the activity of other muscle groups and will help you burn additional calories.

Before You Begin….

Before you begin your bodyweight work out, it is important to thoroughly warm up your muscles. Getting the heart rate elevated and the blood and oxygen flowing through your muscles greatly reduces the chances for injury. If you happen to be running short on time, you always want to cut short the actual workout AND NOT THE WARMUP. You can warm up in a variety of ways such as running in place, riding on a stationary bike for ten minutes, or casually jog up and down stairs. It is important not to overdo it during warmup.

How Often Do I Do This Workout?

Basic bodyweight workouts should be done two to three times weekly, but you don't want to do these circuits on consecutive days. Having a day of rest in between workouts will help your muscles repair quicker and you actually will build muscle during the rest periods after exercise. These bodyweight workouts do not have to be long and tedious; most of these types of basic workout should last from 20-30 minutes. The workouts can also be shorter if you are running low on time. After your workout is complete, it is wise to cool down with some slow stretches.

A Sample Basic Bodyweight Circuit

A basic bodyweight workout for beginners can look like the following:

*Body weight squats (a set of 20)

*Push-ups (a set of 10—can include push-up variations once you get stronger)

*Walking Lunges (a set of 20)

*Dumbbell Rows (a set of 10--you can use milk jugs or other similar household items if you wish)

*Planks and side planks (beginners should try to hold these for at least 15 seconds)

*Jumping Jacks (beginner should aim to do 30 jumping jacks and increase with greater stamina)

Some Things To Keep in Mind...

As you go through this bodyweight workout, there are some things you can incorporate to help you complete your workouts easier as well as make the workouts more challenging and fun. For example, if beginners are having difficulty with the squats or lunges, it is perfectly acceptable to use a chair or other means of support to stabilize yourself until you build strength. The same can also be said for pushups. If you have difficulty in performing a basic push-up, you can start on your knees until you build the strength needed to perform a regular push-up.

In order for any of these exercises to be effective, it is important that you practice proper technique. In order for you to achieve proper technique, there are certain visualization aids that you can employ. For example, when performing squats you want to think of doing a squat as if you were sitting back comfortably in a chair. Try sitting down in a chair and then immediately stand up. If you are able to stand up without having to lean forward, that is how a proper bodyweight squat should feel.

When you perform lunges, it is extremely important that you keep your eyes focused ahead and that your upper body remains vertical. Keeping this proper alignment will help you more effectively engage your core muscles, which are critical to your overall growth in strength and endurance. Additionally, when performing the dumbbell rows, you want to use objects that are heavy enough to provide some form of resistance but aren't so heavy as to cause muscle strain and injury.

Most important of all, bodyweight training (and any type of training for that matter) will be for naught without proper diet and nutrition. You need to be sure that your diet is loaded with fruits and vegetables as well as lean meats and nuts. You also want to focus on eating foods that are natural and whole, and you want to cut out the junk like caffeinated soda, candy and fast food. Diet and nutrition constitutes the bulk of overall health and wellness.

The Best Option for Beginners

For beginners that are looking for an exercise program that is easy to do and follow and doesn't require expensive equipment, gym memberships and potential embarrassment, bodyweight workouts are an excellent way to kick start your commitment to fitness and overall wellness. These exercises can be scaled back to accommodate the beginner, and with the variety of exercises that you can incorporate, your workout routines will never become boring. Bodyweight workouts are also an excellent addition to more formal weight training and the full range of motion these exercises offer can not only help with strength and stamina, they can also help rehabilitate injuries as well.

Before starting any exercise regimen, it is important to consult with your doctor and receive a comprehensive examination. Additionally, your doctor can give you further tips and suggestions regarding which exercises are right for you as you start a program. Start on the path of looking good and feeling your best with bodyweight training.

Thank You Page

I want to personally thank you for reading my book. I hope you found information in this book useful and I would be very grateful if you could leave your honest review about this book. I certainly want to thank you in advance for doing this.

www.ingramcontent.com/pod-product-compliance
Lightning Source LLC
LaVergne TN
LVHW021746060526
838200LV00052B/3504